1

Printed in the United States of America

First Edition June 2014

Library of Congress Cataloguing-in-Publication Data

ISBN-13: 978-1500204730

ISBN-10: 1500204730

Other Books by Mary K. Hukill

Flowers....with Facebook Friends from around the World!

Country Back Roads
4 Volume Book Series
Pictures from Western Kentucky and in Southern Indiana. The Photographer is Eugene Robbins and he travels with wife Grace. She brings the camera.

Community Garden Revolution   2014 Edition
Which comes in the Full Color or Black and White version.

Community Garden Revolution Notes!
2014 Edition

All Books are in the Kindle eBook Version

Coming Soon! Some versions in AudioBooks.

* * *

This is my Story. Hopefully, it will help you. More Families are faced with having to take care of their Family Members than before. It is estimated that in 10 years, it will be an epidemic.

Learn what I've done or faced. It isn't a book of where to go and find services. It is just my account to help others what you may go through, face, and learn to live Life as you go along this Journey. Make of it what it is. Good Luck! I know that others have more Medical challenges to face than I have had and some face less challenges than what I have faced. I help my Mother. It has helped me. I would not do this for anyone else. It is work, hard work, a challenge every day I get up. But, I count it as a God-given Gift to help my Mom. So many others have lost the battle and have lost their parents by their passing. To me, this is a Gift. And, I thank God for every day I have helping my Mom. She helped me many, many times over the years and I couldn't have done it without her.

Thanks! Mom! You deserve the BEST care possible. Today, it is me. I'm the BEST. And, I will do everything I can to be the BEST for you.

Thanks! Mom!

I'm a Caregiver!

Don't Treat me like some Corndog.

By

Mary K. Hukill

...a humorous look at my Journey.

Introduction

Don't treat me like some Corndog. I am a Caregiver. Someone has to help Mom. I didn't grow up thinking this was the way for me, I didn't read it from some Tarot Cards, and, I sure wasn't asked ahead of time by TV Host Art Linkletter if this was going to happen to me. Let alone if it was going to be a part of my Career. I love Children, just didn't want any. I like the idea of being a Grandmother where the kids go after visiting. I'd spoil Grandchildren. So, to end up taking care of a Parent was a Jolt.

This is a lot of work. Sure, you eat well, can sleep somewhere, can enjoy the

Holidays together, watch some TV, see some Movies, and listen to some music together. I'm lucky, my Mom has the skills to play the Piano. Sometimes, when I made sales calls it was kind of cool to have the Piano music in the background. It may have added some high caliber to the calls. Or, it may have ticked some folks off and that is why some didn't do business with me. Either way, I enjoyed it.

I'm not popular with some of the Local politicians and the "Boss Hawg" as some folks like to say in town. Those folks stalked me for Decades and I just kept making Money. When it was more localized situations, they stole Money from what deals they could. I didn't worship the ground they walk on and certainly don't think much of them past a sentence. So, I was punished, 'show her who is boss'. Well, I won in one Big Way, I enjoyed taking care of my Mother who helped me when they Stole my Money. I've been in Financing for 17 years, the Family Business for 20 years and didn't want to take that over, broke my Step-Fathers heart, but, I wasn't too smart in that Field, I believe. He was and very respected. So, right before the Financial Crisis of 2008, I knew the Financial Market was changing but had no idea what was going to happen. Folks, well some bad intentioned Clients, decided not to pay me, some Hotel Deals didn't go as planned and hoped, so, I was Prime to start doing some changes. What I *didn't expect was that God thought the same. So, he presented this option: Take care of your Mother. I was glad, but, didn't know the Journey we'd be taking since I enjoyed my Finance career a lot. It did tick off some of the Stalkers I've had, but, tough. I deserved making my Fees. I closed Millions of Dollars over the years. My local Stalkers didn't want others to know that. I was suppose to be dumb, stupid and not like to make Money. I LOVE and Enjoy making Money. I don't love money—now, that is dumb and stupid. With money you have the Tool to do Great things, help yourself and help others. Sure, you can do the same thing with or without Money. Folks like being paid with Money. It is how it works. I didn't create the World System. But, this gave me a time to regroup, form another Company and see what other Finance Deals were out there. 2009 I had NO Deals, that is a Big Fat ZERO to close. Banks or other Finance folks weren't lending. It was one of the worst years in my Life. I Love making money and I Love my career. So, helping Mom seemed like the time to regroup. I had Food and a Place to Sleep. BUT, taking care of a parent is very time consuming, your money source is squashed til you figure out how to make that work, again, since I don't Qualify for Social Security help, or, Caregiver help. THAT was eye-opening. I'm already Vested for Social Security, but, not the right age. I* want to wait later to draw from that, anyway. I have to make "other" Money to ever think to take it easier when at an elderly age. Folks my age may have to work til we are Dead. I like working, so, I will keep at it in order to have something to do, anyway, as long as I'm Healthy do that.

Well, you keep at it. Who knows what is on God's mind. He has Humor. He wants me to regroup and become a Better person and be the Best I can be. It has been level by level, but, I am feeling better than I have in many decades. Sure, I still have the Stalkers, the crazy "Boss Hawg" folks that are more Crooks than human, but, I keep in there. Revenge is Enjoying Life!

Enough about me. How about why you are here. Lets see what we can do about easing some of your frustrations, your concerns, why me, what is it all about on this Journey, what can I do, is anyone else doing this, what are we doing here, what am I to learn in this stage of Life, etc.

Well, I can ONLY tell you what I've been through. Hope you can gain some insight, tips, or, find that others are going through what you are. Hopefully, we can all learn from each other and keep in there. The Detergent Tide and me have become Great Friends, simpatico, in some situations. I've acquired more new Recipes, gotten some new Kitchen equipment to work with via my Mom's purchases. It has been a journey, and, I'm here to share with you what I've seen and been able to get past, redo, find a way to do, ask others how to do things, and keep your computer on hand for a resource.

Granted, there were many times none of us in the Family knew what was going on, what situations we had to make decisions about, and what was infront of us. We had no other folks for a resource, that we knew, or, even thought. So, Here is my account of what happened in my Life.

*   *   *

Here is my Story and I'm Sticking to it.

Read how I took care of a Parent and survived. You will survive, also. Keep with it, get rest when you can, and eat well is my Story and I'm sticking to it.

To keep up your strength, make lists, a lot of lists, keep Calendars around for Doctor appointments, and, other info, like when to change the mattresses around, yes, you will forget otherwise, and mark down things you need to do that day. Pray a lot. This helps you and your Family Member or Friend. This is what I have done and am doing and hope it gives you some ideas. Sure, there are other such ways of doing things, but, here are some Tips I ran into and what was found to work. Or, not work. Whatever was the actual situation at the time. Don't sweat the small stuff. You will in time, realize that. Life will go on, the World will still revolve, and the E.R. is always available when needed. Don't panic, just react and keep going forward.

Well, here is my Story, and, yes, again, I'm sticking to it.

Enjoy! And Good Luck! And God Bless!

Dedicated to my Mom

Dorothy F. Wolford

And, THANKS! To my Brother for all he does!

Ellis Perry Hukill, III

A "Shout Out" to my Uncle Tommy!

Thomas C. Fullington

In the Beginning!

It started off as a phone call from a Neighbor that my Mom needed help. She had just had a Knee Surgery and thought she could do it all alone from there. All of it.

We all knew differently.

It had to be "her" decision.

We all knew.

She didn't know.

She should have, but, it left her brain.
Well, her conscious.

So, I came over and the rest is History.

I joined the brave new world of the
children taking care of their Parents.
No Manual. No second thoughts. No
going back. No catching a bus to
Nashville, TN, and start a new Life.
This was it.

Was I ready.

Sure, not.

I jumped in head first and it all goes from there.

Sign me UP! I'm ready to do the laundry, fix the food, watch over the bandages, help make sure they Physical Therapy happens, answer the phone, get the mail, dust, the dishes, shine the shoes, take out the Trash, do the snow shoveling, sweep off the sidewalks when storms drop off debris. I'm it, pick up stick. If it is to be done, it is me. Well, Mom does help what she can do and when she is healthy to do.

All I know, is that there is a LOT to do when you are a Caregiver.

Don't treat me like some Corndog.

Folks will stare. Others may not treat you right not knowing your role in things. What I always think is odd is that I have the ear of my Parent. So, if you treat me wrong, what do you think I will be telling my Mom. I deserve respect also for bringing my Mom to your Business, your office, to the Grocery, etc. I don't want you to kiss my behind, just respect me if I have shown you respect also. Treating me otherwise isn't too wise. I help my Parent decide if a good deal is a good deal. When I first started on this Journey, I would be stared out helping a Parent. A year or two later, more people my age were around with their Grandmothers, Mothers, Fathers, whoever. Now, it is becoming very common. It will be the norm in 10 years. Get ready.

I didn't phone in to do this, wave my hand to be picked, or, ask God to do this. I was in Financing for 17 years, the Market changed, I had to change with it, but, some folks decided not to pay me, some Bad Locals (Stalkers and 'Boss Hawg' also) decided to shallack me in the Media from them being paid to do that, evidently, and I am having to keep going forward with a far less money than I made before. I'm working to keep going forward and make the best of it. It is time to regroup, anyway.

Do something for yourself. You aren't dead, yet.

The World isn't going to stop if you take time to see a Movie, do some strolling around Stores and actually see what is there than just buzzing by to keep in a too tight schedule that even Army Commands can't keep up. Go to Church, see a Free Event, have some time going to a Local Meeting, do something to recharge your Life and see what others are doing. Stay current. Read the internet daily.

If you need someone to be there in your place, then, make arrangements with Family, Friends, or, some paid assistance. You have to take care of yourself. You are still alive. You need to rest when possible, eat well, and stop once in a while to take a nap, or, read a book, remember that you are still a human and need some time to embrace that. God put you on the earth to do something. Find some time for that, besides taking care of a parent, a relative, a friend, whoever. Don't cheat yourself.

Peanut Butter can get you from here to there......it won't help about Toilet Paper, though........

Sometimes, you have to do what you have to do. My Mom and I are good planners. So, it has only been once or twice a year that I'd have to run after another ingredient at the Grocery Store that I thought I had but didn't. I'm lucky! One time I thought a bag in the pantry area was Sugar and it wasn't. Oh, well.

Now, if you get too tired of making a Meal, or, who you are taking care of needs something to tide them over, use some good old Cheese and Crackers or some Peanut Butter. For my Mom, that has helped many times when you need to get from here to there. She could snack on other things but we choose to eat healthy items. Yes, we do have Fresh Baked home made items like cookies and sliced banana bread or pumpkin bread around. That helps. I always have various loaves of banana bread or pumpkin bread in the Freezer ahead of time. Peanut Butter is nutritious, it can be economical, if you can call it that in today's prices, but, can be a good item to keep on your shelf.

Toilet Paper, you are on your own. Keep some extra around.

Clean. Be Clean all the time, possible.

You need to realize this is one of the most important things to do: Keep everything Clean that you are cargiving folks touch, sleep on, use, etc. For some coming out of surgery for recovery this can mean the line between life and death. I believe it is that way period. So, learn how to use the Washer and Dryer, get some various Solutions and rags and learn to use the elbow grease. You may think it doesn't matter, but, it can. I believe it does anyway, period. Phases come and go in your caregiving, but, always remember to keep things as clean as possible.

You may have to vacumn the carpet more, sweep the floor more times a day, dust the area more times, wash clothes and items more than you use to, wipe off countertops more often, schedule times to wash the Fan Blades in a room, the tops of the Fridge, wash those sheer curtains more, etc. I mean, be a cleaning machine or hire it. Have the Teenagers help you, have a Group clean up time every so often and attack rooms. This can help Free up some time for the Caregiver who has to do everything else. Be helpful. It does matter Greatly. And, appreciated.

Free Events to go see and do.

Why not go see something FREE in town. That can be a Music event, Art, a Poetry Reading, some Lecture, watch a Demonstration, and, more. You need to do something and get out of the four walls whether it is just you, and, or, the person you are caregiving. Again, always remember, you aren't dead, yet, and certainly don't act like it. If the person can't leave the premises there are a lot of Video tapes, DVD's, or CD's to watch. Set a Special time with them and watch together some Concert, Movie, Sports Event, and enjoy each others company. This may help to provide a stress free way of some down time. Which you need every so often, anyway.

Flowers.

Grow some Flowers. It is Good for the Soul. How many times have we all heard that. It is. Find some colorful seed packages of Flowers to start from scratch or purchase some neat plants and grow in one or various pots. You will need some plant food to help the plants grow, in my Opinion. Have the one you are caregiving help in this process. This helps them have something positive to look at every day and be in the process of caring for it if they can. It just gives them something to look for every day. You choose what you can manage and nothing more. It isn't the Quantity of things, it is the Quality of things.

Container Gardening.

I am a Huge Fan! Of Container Gardenging as that is what my Mom does. Once she left her House of some 30 plus years and moved into a 55 age and above apartment, things changed. She didn't have her Greenhouse anymore. She needed to work on Growing Vegetables to have something positive to do and to nourish her own Soul.

Plus, she looks at how this helps the monthly Grocery bill. It helps. Some years plants grow better than others, but, what FUN!!! it is to eat some Lettuce that day you have Grown from just a seed. WONDERFUL.

When Grocery Shopping may be the next Olympic Sport.

I don't know what it is, but, when I walk into a Grocery store my Brain does a FREEZE until I step right out of the place. When I'm inside, it is to conquer the shelves upon shelves of product that makes me wonder how the stores even sell all of the stuff. I mean, really. Who buys all of this stuff. My Brain feels like all 'smart life' is sucked out and there is a void......infact, I believe there is no man made serum for this condition. It happens all the time. When that electronic two doors open at the front of any Grocery store, some have just one electronic door, they scoop you in push you into their Gigantic maze of shelves, displays, product corna copia that engulfs your Brain that you don't know anything, not going to know what hit you, 'come into my domain my little pretty'…..it is going to be a pure human Jungle to find anything. Zap! 'we have you now, sucker! You have to survive. With my Shopping List in hand and a pen to cross off whatever I could find, ready to replace other items if needed from the lack of finding what was on my List……I'm ready for battle. Now, get your Shopping cart cleaned off with an Alcohol wipe, you are now ready! BLAAHAHAHAHAHAAA!!!!!

Now, the hard part is finding what is on your Shopping list. Yes, you do need to go in there with a Shopping list. It will help.....to a point. Sometimes I have to go round and round the place just to find the Pimento or the Boullion cubes. I've only found the Boullion cubes in one Grocery and not the other, well, I found it one time and haven't seen it after that. I'm sure they sell it, somewhere. Possibly, in the Electronics section. I've not found it yet, is all I can tell you.

For my Mom and me, this is our Scheduled Quality time. We plan out which stores to visit and shop, when to shop, what to purchase there, do we have Coupons, can we use another item to replace what wasn't on the shelf...sure, what I couldn't find. My Mom and I plan out the Grocery Store shopping like McArthur must have done his Missions in WWII. We were relentless to find the best price and where that was in about a 7 store circumference. I was the one to go into battle, well, er, the Grocery Store that were small missions in nature and bring back the goodies. My Mom helped out in larger Missions as she has shopped for years and knows more about bulk pricing or sizes better than me. I like, I buy. She and I have now worked to be more aware of what can be purchased at the smartest price.

Using a Grocery store cart helps a lot of older people, like my Mom, to walk. Get their walking in. Be Stablized when walking. So, allow them to use the Grocery store cart to walk and see something besides their four walls at home. Mom does a lot of reading, but, she needs to walk more and we can do that with going to a store that provides a Shopping cart. Look around. You will see various older folks just walking around with a Shopping cart. They are getting their exercise, getting out of the four walls at home, and seeing what is going on in the World. It helps them with a positive experience and allows them to still feel Human. It allows me to feel Human. I'm for that!

I enjoy seeing what new items are out in the Market, love to see the various Holiday store decorations and the ones that folks can purchase. It keeps me feeling as a Human than a Prisoner. You don't want to feel the ball and chain thing going on. You want to breathe, feel alive, and experience things you use to, although, limited in what and when you can do things. You aren't dead, yet, live what you can do.

Share Special Moments Together.

Mom and enjoy many things together and enjoy things separately. When the Full Moon comes out, or, there are Neighborhood Celebrations that have Fireworks, or, there are Comets flying by.....we try and watch for that. If we remember. Now, most things we do remember and work out a Schedule, meaning put it on a note, and look to experience those things. Sometimes it is just riding to the local Airport and checking out the parked Airplanes or Jets that will be used during an Air Show. We like those kind of things. It is just the cost of the car gas, not any

Tickets, and it is plain all American FUN! to see up close those air craft. Sure, it may be cheesey to some folks, but, we love it. The day has more Excitement, something unique to look forward to, and enjoying something inexpensive together.

Sharing experiences allows for Memories to be made. If you don't do something together, how are you going to share, possibly, learn something new about a subject, and, peel back the layers of what makes that event so awesome. It may be from just being a superb way of even enjoying each others company. Make Memories. Do something together!

When the Neigborhood changes........or, they all have to go to the Nursing Home or live with their Kids.

Things Change. When any of your Neighbors change, die, have to live with their own Children, things will change in your Life. Embrace the change. Sure, some time to realize that something is not going to be the same. Folks can call each other, but, as time goes on folks may not keep in touch. Let things happen as they do. Be there to listen, possibly, show that other new options, and possibly, people may crop up. Let time prevail.

Throw away things. The Smithsonian Museum isn't calling.

Most Families like keeping all their stuff they have collected over the years. Boxes, Bags, tons of just stuff stuck in attics, closets, and garages. Some folks keep stuff in storage areas and pay rent month after month after year after year. WHY!!!

Get rid of it. The Smithsonian Museum isn't more than likely going to call you to display items there. Do it layer by layer and throw away items. Donate to a needy Group, have a rummage sale, give to other Family members, pitch it in the trash. By doing it a bit at a time, you allow the person or persons some time to see that Life goes on, no one is throwing them out, and you need the room. You need to throw away the clutter, the fire hazard, the stuff, period. I have found that doing it layer by layer, it has been more FUN!!! to see what needs to go, help someone sell it at a Rummage Sale versus tripping over anything, having stuff fall down when you are going after another item, and just clearing out things a bit. If you have to ever move or change the arrangements for health care this lessens the load right away. It also is better, I believe, for one's mind health.

It clears out things, lets new possibilities surface, and allows a more clean positive view of where you live and how you live. Hey, that cleaned off shelf allows some older items to be seen for a bit before they take an exit. Enjoy! What you have. Celebrate it. Why are you keeping it all in boxes for someone else to enjoy. Allow yourself to enjoy the memories, or, the colors and brightness those items may present, let Life happen. The other stuff, do you really need it. Really.

Then, why are they stuck in some box.

Learn to let go. Learn to trim down things in your Life. If the House or apartment burned down today, you may not even miss them . Clean it out.

Find items of interest to spark good memories of Life or allow some FUN! time in Life.

Folks like to feel relevant in Life, not matter the age. Donate some time if you can, or, items.

Look at old pictures and change in the Frames you have. I got out all the older framed pictures and hung them where ever I could. One of my Granny's blankets she made is used as a back up on cold nights. Some old pictures she had of painted flowers now hangs in a hallway area and reminds me of her each time I pass by them. We have out old wood pieces that my Step-father made. Good

Memories can be created by the items you have. You don't have to purchase much of anything. Use the items you have. Empty out those attics, those storage places, and use well treasured family items. You will feel good inside. And, you are actually using items instead of storing them and never using them. Use items or give them away.

Buckle Up! your Seatbelts! The Jet taking care of someone is taking OFF!!!

When taking care of someone, you better Buckle Up! each day. The Jet has taken OFF!!! Once you get up to the time you get to bed for the evening.......it is one issue, one situation, one crisis, one thing after the other. Learn to take it in stride, let the small stuff shake off, do one thing at a time, even though you do have to learn to multi-task, and get what you can get done and start all over the next day. If making a List of things to get done helps, then do it. You will keep adding things to the List as the day progresses. Sometimes a List allows you to keep focused on what to accomplish that day and what important things are needing to be done versus what pops up, what needs to be added, why didn't they remind you of adding something to the List, and who says we have time for all of that, Today. You only can live one day at a time and that is what you can only do. Don't fret. It is frustrating to not get all your List done when in Business or working for others you easily did. This is Caregiving and if the US Navy, Airforce, the Army, the US Coast Guard, Secret Service, and who ever could do it, they would. Oh, and THANKS! To all the Men and Women Military Service folks for all you have done and are doing to help keep America FREE. And, to all those Vets out there that have sacrificed so much for our Country. THANKS! Salute.

Bottom line, is that this Caregiving is hard work, the days go by FAST from all that you have to do and work to get done, and, there are many times you get to enjoy what goes on in a day! Those moments you cherish and will treasure. Enjoy! It all, the messy, the dirty, the great FUN!!! you will have doing a job well done. Find satisfaction that you were able to survive it. You will survive it. ONLY if you do take care of yourself in the process. Amen.

Celebrate! The Holidays!

As they come in the course of a year, do Celebrate all the Holidays. This creates memories, it gives everyone the cause to Celebrate and mark the course of the year. I even remember Cinco de May, the fifth day of May each year. Bring out the Flags and place in your front yard, they don't have to be big Flags, the smaller ones on a small wood dowel rod will work, place some Easter eggs in a Basket on a Table if you don't want to get too elaborate, have out some small Christmas trees all decorated, or have a Manger scene sitting on a shelf or table. Learn to actually experience all the Holidays instead of just marking time. We like going through various Retail stores at Christmas to see all the in-store decorations. It is just always amazing what is out in the Marketplace. It is cheap entertainment, but, we have a blast. And, when time, we do go a night or few to see the Christmas Lights. What FUN!

The car keys goes to the one that can drive. The car.

Some families just don't care, is my Opinion. Each family handles when to cut the keys to the car to an older parent. My Grandparents hid it for years. They would get a new car every year, for a bit, because they kept getting in car accidents. We didn't know. It wasn't odd, at the time, since my Great Aunt lived near them and she always had gotten a new car for many years, every year. You expected that when visiting her. My Grandparents were more conservative with their Money and it wasn't odd til they go TWO new cars in one year. Well, my

Uncle drove to their House in another state and decided to give my Grandfather a driving test. Well, the white knuckle drive started. My Uncle isn't Catholic, but, I'm sure he wanted a Rosary in his pocket. My Grandfather drove all over the sidewalks, didn't make a turn too well to turn around going back to the house, when at the house was asked to drive to the carport area down the driveway to the house. My Grandfather hopped over the curb and stopped the car infront of the Front door of the house, instead. On the Front lawn. He gibbly said to my Uncle, who I'm sure was saying Prayers under his breath "How's that". Yes, my Grandfather Flunked the driving test. With flying colors. He even offered to my Uncle to at least have my Grandmother have a set of car keys. Well, Granny was having Alzheimers and that wasn't going to be too helpful, my Uncle luckily thought. My Grandfather tried. The keys went ONLY to the private hired help they had 24 hours a day.

My Mom does real well, but, has her strength times......her hands sometimes on long drives need to be rested and I can tell from her shaking her hands that it is time to step in and drive. She loves to drive. It gets her places. Sometimes, the legs may not have the strength to walk and that is a day she won't be driving. So, it is touch and go with us, at the moment. She loves to ride and go. She did as a Kid and it hasn't subsided. She use to travel down the lane with her Ryder Red Wagon and thought she was something. I'm sure she was a tough gal on a Tricycle, too. Mom is always up for a drive out of town when needed or when she can. We're enjoying the time we can drive. Sure, Mom would rather fly to destinations.

Right now, we're driving, and a Motorcylce is certainly out of the picture. Horses, too.

Good Luck! When you decide when to take the car keys away. Keep your Family member safe and others, too.

Dry Skin Happens.

Help your Parent, Friend, or Family Member with some Cream on their high upper arms, their back, or legs. In the Winter their Feet can get nasty dry. Help them. Plus, it helps massage their feet for a tad and usually helps make them feel good.

Paint some Toenails, or, Massage Feet, put some Lotion or hand cream on their back.

A lot of folks don't have anyone to help them. Offer some time to help a Relative, a Friend, a Neighbor. You may want to show that you they are Human and you understand that.

Also, make sure those Toothbrushes are changed every so often.

What is 'Tall', to begin with, now.

My Mom is 'Tall' to me, no matter the height she is now. After one surgery she started losing inches. Well, enough for us to make Adjustments. First, you start seeing what clothes can fit. Then, how are you going to reach things. The Kitchen was more problematic than anything. Everything that she needed to reach had to be put on the Kitchen counter or the first shelf space in the Kitchen cabinets. We still adjust, but, much closer to what is needed to make her Quality of Life experience a fit. Sure, she can't reach too much in the far lower cabinets so that was the perfect time to clean them out and just put what she needed up front by the Cabinet Door. I can reach the rest. Just like I do in the Supermarket for Mom. She can do eye level pretty good, from there on up I have to help reach the product. I don't mind. It is part of what goes with the caregiving package. My Mom can't reach the Stove Hood Fan or Light, but, sometimes on her tippy toes she can at least turn the Light on. I don't trust her on the Stool too much when alone for balance. My Goal is to not keep too much of that activity happening so I pretty much have everything she needs at the level she can easily reach it. That works in my situation. We did the same thing with the Bathroom and moved around

Towels, items she may need, etc. The rest is 'storage' to her since she can't reach them. Just adjust. Take it in calm and stride since you have to adjust to make it happen.

Make the adjustments needed to fit who you are caregiving, do it matter of factly, as they can't control if they lose inches on their height. It is part of the aging process for most. Several inches for some may be lost, and less for others, but, it is a part of the aging process, keep going forward.

Things can happen with Teeth. Well, Dentures.

My Grandmother was always a Hoot. I think later in Life she knew she was just passing through. She didn't do any Volunteer work once she and Granddaddy retired. They should have. Back then, people didn't live as long as they do now, but, they did. So, they were bored, sometimes.

On one occasion, my Grandparents came to visit and went with my Parents to a Business meeting that was about 4 Hours away and 4 Hours back. Well, they always had a Grand Ole' time when going somewhere together. After about at least an hour going down the Highway, my Grandmother got very serious. Which my Grandmother was a person that liked to laugh and enjoy a good conversation. Finally, my Mom asked why was the matter. Well, my Grandmother was devastated. She sheepishly stated…..mumbled…….'she forgot her bottom teeth'. What? My Mom asked. Granny stated much more confidently "I forgot my Lower Dentures". Oh, oh, my Grandfather thought. "She'll need those to eat".

My Step-father was kind enough and drove all the way back to get her lower Dentures. They laughed all the way back, but, was glad it wasn't something else. You adjust. Life as a caregiver is all about adjusting. If you aren't adjusting every day you get up, someone is either dead or you are. Just take the punches, er, adjustments as best as you can. They are going to happen. Make light of it and you will get through your day much better.

I sometimes write notes before we leave some appointments in a day to make sure what we need, is it near the door on a table by the car keys. Do what you need to do to remember things as the one you are caregiving may distract you, for no apparent reason or that they are just too hyper that day. You have to be in control of your time and thoughts. The other person will help, but, do NOT depend on them. Sometimes it may seem they

are just there going along for the ride.
You are to help, but, know that you
need to also make sure you bring along
what you may need. We keep various
items in the Trunk of the car. Alcohol
wipes are a Great Tool and I like them.
Have enough around for all needs.
This helps you keep folks clean,
surfaces clean, and your hands clean.

Also, when Shopping or going on
errands with the folks you are
caregiving make sure you know where
Restrooms are in stores, places,
events, beaches, etc. You have to
react as fast as you can some days.
Pads for folks may need to be worn.
So, what. You came in the World
doing the same thing.

My Uncle likes to warn folks if there are TWO that you have to take care of, like Mom and Dad, you need to have another person go with you to the Stores or errands. He remembers vividly how he drove my Granny and Granddaddy to the store and was tending to my Grandfather's order and my Granny was no where to be found. She had other ideas. She wondered off in a jiff. My Uncle had to have someone else in the Store watch Granddaddy and he had to tear down aisle by aisle til he found my Granny just taking her time looking at the shelves as she walked past. She was having a time of her Life looking. Enlist some help if it is more than one you have to watch in a Public place.

Candy is good.

My Mom and I enjoy! Eating Candy.
Mom is even better at making it. My
Brother is awesome in making Hard
Candy. My Brother and Step-Mother
are the BEST Caramel Candy Makers.
When it isn't my Brother and Mom
making it. (Family Politics.) (I can sit at
the Thanksgiving Table this year, now.)

Sometimes, you make a batch and give
it away. Mom makes the BEST Fudge
around. Well, my Brother makes the
BEST Peanut Butter Fudge around. I'm
the Taste Tester! YES! I can do that!

These Holiday times, and throughout
the year, Candy brings us together. My
Brother can tell you what Candy

Thermometer is best, and helps regulate what is being cooked in the pan on the Stove. I'm in another room as I'm just the Taste Tester. My Mom and Brother are the Brains in the Kitchen and…….I'm just the Taste Tester. I like it when they are baking in the kitchen as it helps both of them. They spend Quality time together and have a hoot of a time. Mom makes her List about six months ahead of time what she is making folks at Christmas time. During the year, Mom and my Brother Buddy, as we call him, others call him Ellis, and, they plan out how to make whatever it is that I'm to Test Taste, er, make for others and put them into cute little paper bags. When you have projects that folks can do, this helps them think of others, it helps them in a therapy type setting to grow more strength, have some positive experience, and allows them to fell human. Find something to do. It can be scrapbook making, pottery, painting, knitting, wood working as a helper, golf, gardening, cutting up scraps for a Quilt, etc. Allow folks fo become involved in something, if they can. Otherwise, offer to read to them, provide some Music from their Era for them to listen to in the Quiet of the Evening, watch a Movie from their time period of long ago........bring out the Humanity of Folks. You or them are not dead, yet, don't become the walking dead. Live. Live. Live Life.

The check book. Whose is it, anyway.

Work out who pays for what, how much from which party, and how is that paid.

At some point in Life, some folks have to turn over their Book keeping to someone else. Every situation will be different. Have a plan. Make sure the Math is done right, keep the lines of Communication of what is happening, and, treat the other person with the respect they deserve.

Just be sure the transition is done right, fair to the other person, and the Bills are paid.

Write down Notes that later you can actually read.

I can't tell you how often I've tried to keep up with Phone calls and written down folks information and then later looked at the notes and wondered what Arabian or Hispanic person came to write this stuff down. Horrible writing, chicken scratch looks better. It is amazing when I write down the notes that at the time it looks ledgible. Later, who knows what the notes say. Take your time to write down the important stuff. The Doctor's office or the Pharmacy will just have to wait til you write it down properly. Do take the time. Or, learn Arabia or Hispanic language.

Learn to sing, dance, and enjoy each other as the great humans we all are.

Enlist the Parents Friends to call or stop by and break up things. This may also give you some time to do some thinking, some toe nails, paint your toe nails if a Female, heck do them if you are a Male. Make sure that you have some time for yourself every so often. You didn't sign up to allow someone else's life to take over yours, but, it can, and, sometimes quite Quickly.

Christmas Baking can be FUN! even with flour all over the floor.

My Brother and Mom can Bake up a Storm. Infact, that was a Tool I used to help my Mom build up strength from a horrible need for a Surgery recovery. She was actually having to work from ground zero building up her strength. So, I placed a card table in the Living Room….yep, so I had plenty of space to work with….layed down the Tools, the Flour on some wax paper and we went to town baking some Cookies. It was Great Therapy to a waif of a body Mom had at the time. We kept doing this for several batches and several times til she finally wanted to work in the Kitchen. It was miraculous in many ways.

Christmas Baking allows Families to create memories.

Anticipation is good.

You are the caregiver. Believe it or not, you are the one that has to rely on your Quick thinking, experience, the folks needs to decide ahead of time what can or could happen. Anticipation is your Best Friend, also. If they need to bring a Walker or Cane to a large Building that could prove needing some help, then bring it. If you don't use it, so what. But, if you need it and didn't bring it, where would you be in that situation. Who cares if it 'hurts their feelings' or want to state they don't need a cane. Bring it anyway, it is better to be prepared than not. Sure, sometimes I feel like I'm thinking for TWO people and not just for myself. Which can tire someone out. You are the caregiver and you have to think out all possible options of what could happen. Don't trust who you are helping. Denial, them not letting you help them when needed, ego, and other issues can't creep in and won't if you don't let it. You can anticipate situations without them feeling less than human. Just mention you are doing or bringing items of help to be sure you don't need them, even when you know you may. Anticipation will cut down problems that may happen later and sure makes my mind at ease. Hope it helps you and your Family.

Quality time for yourself.

You need to find some time every day for yourself. I know it is hard. I'm there, been there, know it. You need to unwind, go over the day, get ready for the next day's schedule.

You need to find some time in each day to meditate, think out things, take a nap, read a book that you like, write some notes to some Friends or Relatives, get your Hair done, get a Massage, go to the Spa, do something for you. It will matter. If you don't take care of "YOU" how can you take care of anyone else. They are depending on you and you need to know that you need to watch after yourself also.

I like a Good cup of Tea later at night and just sit for a bit, when there is something new to eat that is tasty and delicious I may sit down with some Coffee and nourish myself with a good food item. I may go take a walk. There are neat store items to look at and see what is going on in the World. Stroll along some Hardware stores and look at the Flowers along the shelves. Look at some pottery being done. Notice I didn't say go out and spend Money. But, if you like to shop and can afford to do so, that is what you need to do. Take your mind off of caregiving and take care of yourself.

Nap.

My Goodness. Who doesn't like a good nap every so often. Whether it is every day or every so often, learn that taking a nap is a good thing. If your folks you are looking after do it why don't you take a nap when they do. I work on things when my Mom takes a nap, and, sometimes I rest my eyes for 15 or 20 minutes. During some news I may take a 30 minute nap and be ready for Show number 2 that day is how I look at things. The second part of the Day caregiving. For us the Evening is better, it flows better and I can get a lot of my work done. The daytime is what it is and what happens, in our Household. I use to use the Morning for making Deals and working to make more Sales Calls. That doesn't happen much for me, but, we are working to carve out a day or two a week to do that. I appreciate that. Otherwise, I'm stuck with just afternoon time to do the important part of my Work. Whether making Sales Calls or writing Books, the afternoon is when I can reach folks on the phone in 3 time Zones, which I call them all.

Naps are Great at any age. I did it when as a Child, when visiting with my Grandparents, and do it Today. I think a body does need to rest every so often. I'm not ashamed to state such. Naps are good to do when possible.

Travel.

When you can that may be a Good Thing for you and the ones you help. If they can Travel. If not bring the World to them and watch Slides, Films, Movies from the Local Library and see places. Make it an Italian night and have some great eats that are of Italian nature and watch some Travel bits.

If you can Travel remember to add in more Alcohol wipes, snacks that are helpful, pack in some yogurt and nuts, bring all the Medicines needed, and have a List of Doctors and phone numbers handy if ever needed. The main goal is to enjoy each others company and have some FUN!!!

Don't leave the House or Apartment for Errands until you are ready.

It is too easy to leave the premises for doing errands and to not be ready. Who you are caregiving can distract you more than you know. And, sometimes they just don't realize or want to realize you need to have your act together.

I have forgotten to bring my Drivers License, I've forgotten to bring some Documents needed for an appointment, there is the need to bring the right set of keys to open a Lock Box or storage unit, there are hundreds of other things that I've now learned to write down notes of what is needed for appointments and errands. You are the caregiver and need to pause before leaving the premises that everything is ready to do. I have found that my Mom is ready to go when she feels good and she is often at the door even before we're ready to leave. She is ready and wanting to do something, now. So, keep your cool, make sure you are really ready to go and THEN go out the door. If you have to drive back, so what. Make sure all things that need to be turned off is off. Make sure that you have everything you need to make your appointments or errands a success.

Call others and chat.

I call people on the phone just about every day. Sales calls require either contacting folks by email or being on the phone. Most email, at first.

Otherwise, I'm not on the Phone. I'm not one for talking, chatting on the phone. Mom likes to call and talk to her Friends. She likes it when someone calls her, especially at the Holiday time. I think most folks like to know that someone is thinking of them and acknowledges that they are significant to them. If you have some older relatives or friends, do call them. I'm sure they will appreciate that you even thought of them. Take the time.

I met Joel Olsteen earlier, but, Church TV for sure was going to be my way of Praising Jesus.

He never looked so Good. Sure, I met Joel Olsteen on TV before helping my Mom. Little did I know that he'd be the one to provide some Church Service moment when taking care of a Parent. Everyone worships differently. Find a way to keep it going. Hey, I use to go to a Catholic Church for Ten years and I'm a Protestant. So, finding the good word, has been interesting, to say the least, but, you have to find it. You need the mental vacation, you need to get yourself right with God, if that is the way you live Life, and you need the time to reflect, think, and see what path is the best for your life. Learn to meditate, have some time to think, and just stop for a moment while the World zips by you fast. Stop once in a while. Stop and smell the Roses. Stop and take it all in. Take time to reflect.

Zip into something dazzling to wear even going to the Pharmacy.

There are only so many hours in a day. You are inside most of the time, when you have the Opportunity to go out and do errands, then, dress up. You need to do that for yourself. Everyone else can look sloppy, but, you need some uplifting moments. Dress up and feel good about yourself. You need those moments. You need to feel good and look good. Get your Hair done every so often. Get a Massage or go to a Spa. I like getting a neat desert that we wouldn't take the time to make. Or, purchase a more expensive piece of meat and grill out. But, time to time, do Dress up. This will help you feel better and you need to know that you feel value, you have value, and that you deserve to be treated that you have value. My Family likes to go to our area Walgreens where the Staff is top notch, we've grown with them from job to job, and new careers, to what phases they are in their lives. We become a part of them and they of us.

You need that in your Life. To feel, still, a part of the Human race.

Dress up! Hey, you never know if you find your next career, your next help of some particular need, or, your next person of special interest. Do it for yourself.

Let the small stuff Roll.

Life is too short. Enjoy! Laugh, cry, be with others, share, and live Life.

Don't strive to win all the arguments. Sometimes you just have to let it roll.

Don't think you have to answer all Questions since some of them may not make any difference anyway. Or, even make any sense. Enjoy the time you have with folks you are a Caregiver.

Really, is it that necessary to be 'right' when you may very well be wrong.

Memory....

I'm telling you, for me, there are many Lists that are made. It has been done for Decades, but, when you have to keep up with someone else, you need to keep a List of things to do, what needs to be done, where are you going and when. Your Calendar is your BEST friend. Your Lists will keep things flowing and going. Don't pride yourself on what you keep forgetting. Write out any and all Lists and keep things going forward.

Social Security for Caregivers

$3,000 a year for those that Qualify is not enough, in my Opinion. I didn't Qualify. And, at the time I was still calling on Financing Sales calls before writing Books. I had something to do while inbetween tasks helping a Parent. The initial Goal was to make money. I wanted to get back making what I could and did make, and, grow from there. When I got to Projects that were 5 digit Commissions, which I've made in the past, and, then at 6 digit and 7 digit Commissions that is where the Local politics broke in and stole those opportunities. I live in a town that has some issues and won two years in a row the top ten in "Most Miserable Cities" in America. We also won the top spot of "The Most Obese City in the Nation" one year in this time frame. The United States should look at Healthcare more and consider making this Social Security payment of $3,000 a year higher for those who do stay with their Parents and take care of them---or, keep paying more on Medicare and Medicaid. Good Health care, with or without a Doctor initiated Nurse or Physical Therapy aid costs money. Where are the savings and where can it be done more efficiently.

Bingo or Cards.

For some folks, going to Bingo or Cards allows them to have some Friends or mutual people to enjoy life together. Whatever can work, do it. If it is a Chess Club, or, Shuffle Board, why not. Hey, if a Parent likes Pool, doing Ping Pong, Ballroom Dancing, let them do it. If they can. This gives them some enjoyment, some time with others, possibly, some time you can do other things, and allows them to have some Fun!

Your Parent is still alive and wants to have some outlet. Let it be.

DWTS.....Cha, Cha, Cha!

Well, the TV Show 'Dancing with the Stars' has certainly been a Popular and Favorite past time with Mom and her Friends. They are on the phone during the Commercials with their comments on the attire, the hair, the Dancing, the comments, whatever strikes their fancy. They have hit all the cylinders on this show. The phone lines light up like a Christmas tree, especially when controversy happens. This is a Show they all enjoy, Together. My Brother writes up, each year, a several page Program for them, with pictures and details of the various Dancers, and presents it to each Lady. They love the attention, it makes it FUN! for the Ladies to feel they are participating in something with others, and they get to share their various opinions with others without any Judgement. One of Mom's Friends is 90 this year and she even has Ledger Sheets to keep up with each Dancing Team. This helps her mind keep sharp, she loves numbers anyway, and she even asks Mom what past scores were listed to keep her Ledger Sheets accurate. She feels this allows her to come up with the possible Winner, in the end. She is usually right, but, doesn't the TV Show also show the Totals as we go along. Anyway, she has also watched the TV Show called 'The Bachelor' for many years, she's never been married, and at the age of 90 years, she has grown tired of it. We don't know the reason, she just was not watching it this year, anymore.

And, when the TV Show 'Dancing with the Stars' made various changes to the Show over the years, or, added Dancers, well 'dancers' to the show that year, the Ladies would all voice their Opinion like it was watching the Super Bowl and all the games that added up to that. They were definitely Quarterbacks and steering the Show how they saw it. The Ladies are into the Show, it gives them something positive to watch, and remember a day long ago when folks actually danced arm in arm. And, with music they understood. Oh, yeah, and words they knew and sang. Ole'.

For a moment, the Ladies, and Mom,
could relive what they knew, in a
World constantly changing.

The Safe Place. We hid it at the Safe Place. Where is the Safe Place.

When my Mom came back from her trips in Europe, she got off the plane and then asked, "Mary, where did you put my Jewelry. I am missing my Pearl Necklace, or, it was some other type thing. I stated "I didn't go on the Trip with you, how would I know". So, we hunted til we finally found, whatever it was we were looking for, in a suitcase or coat pocket. It was just about every Trip. I didn't sweat it. I pretty much felt we'd find whatever was lost.

At one time when my Mom had an extended stay at the Hospital, I had to be there every so often, come back to her place and call a list of her Friends or family members. Well, it did concern us to hide things so that we felt that if someone broke into her apartment that they wouldn't find any valuables. That was time for a Bank lock box. For me, some Family Treasures are the very keep sakes others may slough off as just excess. I don't. My Art work from Grade School, some Letters or Cards from Family and Friends since 1976 I keep as ways to tell of milestones or of memories of folks still alive or not.

In my case, I placed some well used Recipes that Mom liked into a bag and placed them in 'safe place'. Which I should know by now that those 'safe places' are never remembered right off. And, that I should write down where things are placed in a 'safe place'. Mom and I have spent a lot of time searching for things, files, information sheets because we placed them in a 'safe place' instead of the usual place. Well, I did that to these Family Recipes. I didn't think about them snuggly hidden, until after my Mom was Finally released from the Hospital and she wanted to make something from that Group of Recipes. And, I think she just wanted to reconnect with them. Well, wouldn't you know....I didn't remember where I placed them in a 'safe place' ......and was scorned....boy, Mom was mad. Where was her cherished Recipes........I always put her things where they don't belong. Finally, I did find them......I told her that I hid what I treasured most and placed them in a 'safe place' for her. The Treasured Recipes was one of those things. Well, Mom, then understood she went overboard and just Quietly took the folders of recipes in a bag I hid and she went over them like long lost Treasures that they were. The Recipes span a lot of living Life. And, we love thinking of all the wonderful moments those Recipes mean to us. Just this past year, we Celebrated the Holidays with various Neighbors and made an old Treasured Hot Punch, filled the Sterling Sivler pitcher up with that, made some Fresh Great Tasting small Biscuits with that, with butter oozing, and served it to the folks with Christmas decorations on a Silver tray. It was FUN! It was the last time to do that as 2 Neighbors have just now left. One left town Today to move to Minnesota and a wife and husband have had to live at a Nursing Home. So, we're glad we did that. Memories doing FUN! things like that broaden your Life, allow you to bring Cheer! To others, and gives you a chance to reach out. We even served two Nurses to the elderly couple and they LOVED being able to share with us. It was our Honor, to Mom and me.

I treasure my Mom's, Granny's, and, anyone else's cherished Treasured Recipes. It is what Life is about. Money comes and goes, but, to have these wonderful Memories of what some of the Recipes represent, is Priceless. Feel Good Goodness, all throughout.

The Computer.

Well, my Mom is thinking about purchasing a Kindle HD. She has done a keyboard for emails, then a Laptop, and, now thinking about the Kindle HD to use when travelling and at her reading area, I often call the Command Center. She does paperwork and the Budget from that same area. My Mom reads a Book a day, usually. She has read a Book on the Kindle and will take a class when she purchases it at the Library which will be FREE. My Brother has been instructed he is taking the Kindle class also, with Mom, so that he can be a Reference center.
He's excited, not. But, he will help his

Mom. I'm sure the Cyber Industry won't be ready when Mom hits the Internet. But, she will catch on, fine, and, she will read more from it than she realizes, in my Opinion. This will help her read better from the light the screen emits and to keep her mind sharp. Do find ways to keep your folks sharp with puzzles, soduku, and, other ways to allow more thinking processes to happen. If an etch-a-sketch will help, hey, go for it. Mom respects the Rubic cube, but, only my Brother can actually figure that out. She doesn't want it around, but, does have Dominos and some Board Games. She likes cards, but, not around anyone that plays what she knows, anymore.

Do find ways to keep folks minds working and solving situations.

I often wonder how my Granny and Granddaddy from either side of the Family would do with Computers. They were alive when Computers were just coming on the scene. And, Cell Phones were just hitting the market the size of a landline phone or larger. At this time in Life, the remarkable achievements of Technology would astound them. I'm sure they would embrace the changes, or, like others just don't pay attention to them. I'd like to think they'd embrace the changes.

Old Geezer.

Mom and some of her Friends like to check out the other Species, but, not interested to marry someone else. They want to live their lives how they do and anything else isn't on the Table. They've been there, done that.

Well, one guy particularly known by several of the Ladies they call "Old Geezer". He's in his 80's and he is on the prowl. Really. Sometimes the grabs. You have to not be around him, stay clear, and run the other way if he comes your way. He likes the Ladies. He use to be a Pastor, but, God gave him the need to be around the Ladies. One time, his Daughter went to a

Bingo game to 'play' and then kept asking the Ladies in the audience, one by one, by one….if anyone wanted to go dating her Father. The gal had to also watch over her Parent, but, at the time, it wasn't on her Schedule, lets say. Well, the Management of the Apartments, for the 55 and above, told the Daughter to stop the soliciting. The Ladies may have not liked the merchandise, or, just wanted to keep single. Some folks didn't want to be around clinging men. Or, want to share their Money with them. Mom let the guy know that she ran 3 Corporations at one time and another man wasn't in the picture, anymore. She liked her FREE time and not having to watch after, wash after, or have to do what the man wanted to do than what she all the time wanted to do. The Lady that lives next door to the 'Old Geezer' owned several Businesses in her Life and still owns two that provides money for her to live how she likes. She is Happy there isn't another man in her Life. Some Men, they just want you to look after them. Not sure why. They aren't that special. Some are even needy. Clingy. Old Geezer just hasn't ever come around to the idea that other Ladies just don't want to mess with him. He's not gotten the message. Tough.

Now, no matter the age, dating is tough. And, evidently it is tough on the older Ladies, also. The same Lady just told Mom that all she has found is Men that at the 3rd date want to know "is it time for Sex, yet". The Lady just says, "No", gets up from the Table and says "Goodbye". You see, some Ladies, who have their own Money, just don't want to do what the "man" wants to do. And, when they are older, well, it really is important to be able to walk away and just do what you want to do.

I'd rather live that kind of Life.

Dine with a Great Menu.

If you have a limited knowledge of what to fix for Lunch or Dinner, learn some new Recipes. You are more than likely stuck at Home and you are now the new "Chef" to make something edible for meals. Do create new ideas, bring in the fool proof menu items, but, do work on the meal plans you can afford and can fix. When you burn items, keep it going and make something new. Don't get mad. Just keep it flowing. Make it look like you know what you are doing. Sometimes you won't know. Just allow yourself to make mistakes, throw away food that just won't cut it….sometimes that can be the meat, also, and keep things flowing.

This is the time you can sit down, finally, and eat something that hopefully will taste Good. I've had my Mom get out the Sterling Silver flatware and we eat elegantly every meal. Even Pancakes with Sterling Silver has some zazz. It is in the Cherry wood chest, why not use them. They are just sitting there. We even use the 70 plus years Crystal dishes every so often. Why, not. They are just sitting there. Again, Pancakes taste pretty Good on them. They look outstanding and we've not even eaten. Liven things up. You aren't possibly entertaining folks like you use to, so, why not enjoy all the finery you have. If you use some nice Tablecloths it can liven up your Table. Live. Use the stuff. It is all there sitting on the shelves. Use it. If you don't, we believe, why let someone when you die. What is that! Use it. Get to those shelves and use it or get rid of it. Get rid of what thing you don't use, have the need to use, or, will ever use. What are you really keeping it for. If a Tornado came through your house, you will have lost it, anyway. Learn to give things up. Learn to become more lean. Use what you have, or, get rid of it. Donate it, give it away, or sell it for pennies on the Dollar. Get rid of it.

There are a lot of Food TV Shows to find new recipe ideas. Sometimes during Lunch we watch part or most of "The Chew". PBS TV has some Great

Shows and new food preparation ideas. Be open to new thoughts about Food, new possible ways to Grill Vegetables and what you can do with Fruits. Folks are always coming up with new cooking, baking, and grilling ideas. Be open to them and try it out! Hey, you can order Pizza if you burn anything or just make a Sandwich.

Aways enjoy what you eat. Learn that it doesn't matter if you have steak, it is the company you have. Make all meals shine in some way. Magic.

Take time to Order Pizza once in a while.

Once in a while you have to crash. Take time off from the Kitchen. I like preparing the Thanksgiving Meal the day ahead and refrigerate. Most of the Meal can be done that day.

When the Wednesday afternoon hits, I order a Pizza and pick it up. The BEST money spent in the course of a year. Well, one the best.

Make a Schedule for others to help.

Reach out to others. Sometimes, you may need help. Possibly, you have a meeting to attend, a Doctor's appointment that is for you, you need some time to just walk around in a store to unwind, or, other needs. Reach out to others. Reaching out is for the strong for they realize they need the extra help. To be weak, is to not reach out. And, in time that will catch up with you in Health, in Money, in Food, in other ways that you won't like, or, need to have to handle also.

Be strong. Ask others to help and just state what the need is so they can.

Take on the hard stuff like losing weight. Infact, do it together! Who doesn't need to lose a few pounds.

For my Mom, her Health plan is to lose weight. This will help her superb Health, but, also possibly keep us from having to do any more procedures or surgeries. This helps her Heart. There are so many other benefits. So, I stated that I have to lose some weight, which I do. Well, we're on the weight losing trail and doing a pretty good job at it. Plus, it helps my Mom realize that she isn't doing this alone. There is no shame, no hardship in meal planning, and, she is more accountable. We both shop at the

Grocery Store with more intent to purchase the best possible food to help us on our Goal to lose weight. The Selections are more colorful, a more diverse menu, and lots of FUN! to eat as we know this will help our bodies be more healthy. Good Nutrition has always been a forefront of my Mom when she prepared meals. Now, we both have lazor beam thoughts how we can eat better, what will fuel the body better, and what foods will help us.

Yogurt is my Friend. We both eat it every day to keep our Body System in good shape. My Mom likes nuts of every type and eats more fiber. We've always eaten Fruits and Vegetables and that have helped us over the years. Now, we eat more and have a better varied food preparation for the ingredients. It is far more FUN! to prepare and plate. Sure, some days you are too tired to care...but, you have to keep at it. Fix something simple that meal. Sandwiches, soups, salads, can be your good best friend.

Once a week, we like Pancake day that allows a treat for my Mom and I place Chocolate Chips in them. I eat a different meal, but, we both have Scrambled eggs with what we eat. Also, have a neat FUN! expected meal once a week. I like to prepare a GOOD meal at Sunday Dinner. This kinds of gets us ready for the upcoming week.

When you aren't sure make a Batch of Brownies.

Living by myself, for years, when it would Snow I liked eating Fresh baked Brownies as a Treat and watch outside the Window the Snow adding up. Sometimes, I even made Popcorn if it was a bigger Snow expected. If a Movie was on TV or around to watch that was a perfect evening to unwind. Even better if there was too much Snow to worry about the Traffic the next morning and working from where I lived.

Well, when you are living with someone else, you can bake the Treats for someone else. Now, some times,

I'd bake other items like Sweet Cinnamon Rolls, Banana or Pumpkin Bread. But, Brownies pretty much was the rule of order. Being in the lower Midwest, we didn't get much snow. The Climate Change has allowed us to have more, so, I bake various food items to keep things FRESH in what is eaten.

And, sometimes, you just have to unwind, realize the day went as it did, and there is nothing you can do about it. Just unwind. Things Happen. Make a batch of Brownies.

Who says you have to share. Sure, you will. You like to give. You are a caregiver. But, do remember to have some yourself. They will taste WONDERFUL.

Your perspective may change, you will have some time to think situations out better, possibly, differently, and you will be less stressed. You have to find a way to shut down stress, every so often. If you don't, your body will. You don't want to be sick. You are a Caregiver and you are needed. You are important. Work to keep as healthy as you can. But, do indulge in something that will help you feel Good about Life. We all need to feel Good that we're here in the World. Some may scoff, and want you to only eat something healthy, but, a good batch of Brownies may help! Sometimes, you have to splurge and have something tasty Chocolate Good.   Enjoy!

What can I tell you.

There isn't much more I know to tell you. Every person will meet the challenges and the Journey differently. But, some of the real basics are the same. If you can't pay for the Service, you can do what I'm doing. It is tiring, I would NOT do this for anyone else, and it has allowed more time with my Mom. Otherwise, I'd be working a lot since I enjoy working. I do work on my Books and dabble with Financing as it is my Career. I enjoy writing my Books as a good creative outlet. And, if it helps even just one person, then, I've done my Job. I didn't help Mom with some Manual, didn't have a clue what to do some days and improvised, I still improvise, and most days it worked out. For the Days that are long, nasty, mean, hard to get through, just keep at it. Tomorrow is another day. Keep in there. You were helped as a Child and Student. Possibly, you were helped as an Adult. This is YOUR time to give back and do it with grace, with manners, and with confidence. It does matter. And, how you want to be treated is how you treat the one you are caregiving. At least at the end of the Day you know you did your BEST and that is all that matters. Make sure you make them King or Queen and know that God is watching. Sometimes you have to pray for help to make things happen and get through them. God is there. Pray.

You will survive. Ask for help when you need it. Accept help when it comes and from where it comes.   You can't do it all by yourself. I'm glad to help my Mom. It is a Gift. God given. Now, I have to make sure that I did it correctly, brilliantly, the BEST I can do, and do it with grace. And, when you can have some FUN!!! doing it, that is icing on the cake.

Cheers! And, Good Luck!

A Mom read.

And, a Mom Approved Book.

THANKS! Mom!

The End.

Mary K. Hukill lives in the Midwest, of the USA.

I love Gardening, watching on TV Golf, Formula One car racing, The Kentucky Derby, the Indianapolis 500, Comedies, and a Good Movie when it comes along.

Donate to my Favorite Organization the *American Community Garden Association.* And, Start a Community Garden where you live, work, or play. THANKS!

Email: flowersbookseries@gmail.com

www.ingramcontent.com/pod-product-compliance
Lightning Source LLC
Chambersburg PA
CBHW021408170526
45164CB00002B/561